Caregiving
and Understanding Respite

Caregiving
and Understanding Respite

Janice Williams, RN

Dedication

I dedicate this book to my mother, father, family members and all the beautiful family caregivers that I have met over the last ten years.

My Testimony

God proved that He was in control of everything that we faced as we cared for our father. Sitting here remembering like it was yesterday; about how God got my attention during my caregiving journey. I found myself focusing on all the negative things. I was exhausted and stretched in every way possible. I had taken off work frequently. It seemed like there was not enough help. I was in a new place and trying to feel my way through. I was drained and empty.

I was not caring for my father all alone. There were other family members involved in the caregiving. Through the grace of God, we were able to get some others to help us. But it was still very exhausting and stressful.

I just remember feeling overwhelmed and frustrated. Then one day God began to speak to me. He said, "Do you want The Blessing?" Initially, I dismissed what I thought I heard. He spoke loudly again and said, "Janice, do you want the blessing?" I answered him back and said, "Yes Lord, I want the Blessing." At the time I did not know what that meant. I just said "YES." I realized He was trying to get my attention to redirect my focus to what was really important. Which was ensure my father's care needs were addressed and he was comfortable.

You see family caregivers really do go through a lot of things. This role can be very emotionally and physically draining but we cannot only be directed by our emotions. I am saying this because some of the things you will go through on this journey only God can fix. That's exactly what He was trying to tell me. If my focus remained on everything else, especially the negatives, I would miss what He was doing in this situation.

I am telling you, please stop focusing on everything that is negative or does not feel good now. If you don't, you're going to burn out and use all your energy on things that you can't change. When God redirected my thinking, I started to see things differently, not in frustration and not focusing on everything else at once. My focus was redirected to the true care my father needed in his last days.

My dad was not very affectionate. He was a very hard worker and very firm in some of his ways. He never really told me that he loved me even though I knew he did. He took care of us and provided us with food, a roof over our heads, and other things.

One day, I got up the courage to talk to my father about getting him some more help with his daily living activities. I asked him what he wanted us to do for him and how he wanted us to care for him. He told me, even as sick as he was, that there was "no need to be overly concerned because I'm going to beat this thing. I'm going to get better. Thank you, but I won't need all the help that you are talking about." My dad was very independent, even until the end. He never really accepted that he needed some help.

I am so grateful to God. Looking back now I see that if God had not redirected my thinking, I would have missed some of the greatest moments with my dad. After the conversation above with my dad regarding his needs, I finally got the courage to tell my dad that I loved him. His immediate response was that "I Love You Back!" I was like, WOWWWWW. Thank You Lord!!!!!!!!!!!!!!

You see, because God redirected me (and I listened), I got something that I never had before, which was hearing my dad say he loved me. I'm so grateful to God for the experience of being able to provide care to my dad in his last days. The caregiver role is a very hard job when caring for a loved one due to our emotional connection to that individual. However, I want you to know that there is a blessing in it. We all know that we're blessed, and that God is good, but there's another level of blessing that comes out of the caregiving role. I'm redirecting you right now in this book because there's a blessing in being a caregiver.

Caregiver's Respite

After my father died, I saw caregivers were everywhere. I realized family caregivers were in my neighborhood, at church, and on the job. I began to think about the people I never saw again and found out it was because they were caring for their loved ones. I ask individuals all the time, "Do you know of anyone who takes care of their sick family member or love one?" When I ask this question, some have replied yes, they know someone who is a caregiver. Many times they will say no, I don't know anyone. I always tell them that if you think for a few minutes someone will come to mind who is a family caregiver.

As a nurse working in the hospital, I remember seeing a caregiver sitting with her husband one day. I tried to give her husband the medicine ordered by his doctor. He would not take it. This caregiver told me exactly what to do to get him to take the medicine. When I did just what she said, he took it just like she said. I went home after my shift and came back the next day and the same caregiver was there at her husband's side again. She did not get a break, but I did.

God inspired me to start Caregiver's Respite so family caregivers can get a break. Caregivers need a soft place to land. When you take a break (or respite), you can get some rest and rejuvenation. You get a chance to release emotions and stress. Also, you can get information to equip yourself for the situation you will be returning to. Use this strategy to increase your opportunity to become a successful caregiver. That is what I want to leave with you. Your success is not measured by what you feel. Your success comes through the strategy of Respite.

I often tell people we cannot take you out of your caregiving situation, but if you get a break, you can make it. Don't give up and please get your breaks!

CONTENTS

respite • renue • relief • recess • reprieve • rest • breather • breathing space • downtime • hiatus • interruption • lay-off • letup • lull • recess • relaxation • relief • reprieve • truce • break • time • adjournment • breath • cessation • ten • deferment • delay • deliverance • discharge • ease • exculpation • five • forgiveness • halt • immunity • intermission • interval • leisure • pardon • release • stop • postponement • protraction • rest • stay • coffee break • time out • renue • relief • recess • reprieve • rest • respite • breather • breathing space • downtime • hiatus • interruption • layoff • letup • lull • cessation • ten • deferment • delay • deliverance • discharge • ease • recess • relaxation • relief • reprieve • truce • break • time • adjournment • breath • cessation • ten • deferment • delay • deliverance • discharge • ease • exculpation • five • forgiveness • halt • immunity • intermission • interval • leisure • pardon • release • stop • postponement • protraction • rest • stay • coffee break • time out • renue • relief • recess • reprieve • rest • respite • breather • breathing space • downtime • hiatus • interruption • layoff • letup • lull • recess • relaxation • relief • reprieve • truce • break • time • adjournment • breath • cessation • ten • deferment • delay • deliverance • discharge • ease • exculpation • five • forgiveness • halt • immunity • intermission • interval • leisure • pardon • release • stop • postponement • protraction • rest • stay • coffee break • time out • renue • relief • recess • reprieve • rest • respite • breather • breathing space • downtime • hiatus • interruption • layoff • letup • lull • cessation • ten • deferment • delay • deliverance • discharge • ease • recess • relaxation • relief • reprieve • truce • break • time • adjournment • breath • cessation • ten • deferment • delay • deliverance • discharge • ease • exculpation • five • forgiveness • halt • immunity • intermission • interval • leisure • pardon • release • stop • postponement • protraction • cessation • ten • deferment • delay • deliverance • discharge • ease • rest • stay • coffee break • time out • lull • reprieve • break • renue • relief • recess • reprieve • rest • respite

CHAPTER ONE

Wakeup Call

◇◇◇◇◇◇◇

Preparing Our Caregivers to Care

According to AARP[1], ten thousand (10,000) people turn 65 every day. People over 65 are now living longer. One reason is that during their lifetime, medications and treatments have greatly improved.

If you are like I was, you might have an aging parent who does not need a lot of assistance with their activities of daily living. My father was very self-sufficient and because of that I did not get overly involved in his day-to-day routines. Many of us may call and check on our loved ones while missing out on the small details of their daily needs or we may not be as involved.

My dad told me what he needed (if he needed anything) and I would do it. Even that happened very sparingly because he cooked his own food, went to the grocery store, took his own medication, and took himself to the doctor. While talking to him on the phone one day, he told me about his extravagant breakfast that he was preparing: fried eggs, grits, toast, and maybe even sausage! My dad loved breakfast! When he told me all those things, something came to mind that made me feel like I needed to check on him right then. So, I went over to his house. When I got there, he had made that breakfast, but he was sitting on his bed eating out of the pots he cooked in. It appeared that he did not have enough strength to serve it to himself as he usually did. I began to pay closer attention to him from that point on.

My parents were very private people. If they knew how much we shared on Social Media now, they would be livid. Like most people of their generation, they believed that there were certain conversations and topics their children (no matter our ages) should not be privy too. It was none of our concern even when it really should have been. I made it my responsibility from that day on to fill in the blanks that would help me take care of him even when he wasn't volunteering information. I listened and heard what he said but evaluated everything he did.

Family members and I became the caregivers to my father. I think by that point, I had convinced myself that he would live and take care of himself forever. He was sharp and still had his right mind, even at 89. Although, I was in denial for a short period of time. The truth is we can't ignore the fact that our parents will eventually age and may require more assistance during the aging process. We can't reasonably expect them to suddenly say that they need help, they need us to check on them because they get dizzy sometimes, or they need help plating their breakfast. However, we can pay closer attention to details by observing where they are and how they are functioning in their routines.

I have been a registered nurse for many years providing direct patient care. This care includes personal care, administering medications, performing nursing procedures/treatments, communicating with doctors, and educating patients and family members on their health care needs.

As a professional nurse, I've always had and continue to have empathy for the patients and family members (caregivers). Until I became a caregiver for a family member myself, I had no idea of what they actual went through once they were at home on their own. I was suddenly thrust out of my nurse's role into the caregiver role, and I felt like I had no idea what I was doing. Working in the medical field did not automatically make me a caregiver for a family member.

Caregiving truly changes your life. It will test you. It will bring out your strengths and shines the light on your frailties. Caregiving will make you strong, but first you will recognize you are not as strong as you thought. It was not until I started caregiving for my father that I realized that others had been doing it as well. I want you to know now that others are going through similar challenges and have a wealth of knowledge to share with you. We want you to be prepared for your journey through caregiving, even when you feel like you have no idea what you're doing. We are here for you. We want to see you strong and confident. We want you to feel like you can make it **and the first step is Respite**.

Understanding Respite

Respite means a period of delay or a break. Other words for respite are relief, rest, interval, interlude, time out, or pause. Respite is an opportunity for a caregiver to pause so that they can have the chance to care for themselves and decide what to do next. Respite creates a breathing space. It also gives you a chance to not go past fatigue, which is the intensity that comes when you regularly give or pour out in difficult situations. It gives you a short time away so you can continue to assist your loved ones in all the duties necessary for their care.

Many of you reading this book may not even want respite or feel like you need it. You may be so focused on your duty as a caregiver that you don't realize that this job comes with burdens. A burden is a heavy load that can cause a hardship or distress. The responsibility of caregiving is a heavy load that will cause stress - both emotional and physical - and can lead to fatigue. This type of load can crush a caregiver under its weight and leave them tired, lonely, anxious, or even depressed without a break.

◇◇◇◇◇◇◇◇◇◇◇◇◇◇◇◇◇◇◇◇◇◇◇◇◇◇◇◇◇◇◇◇◇◇◇

We can't take you out of your caregiving situation, but with a break, you can make it through it.

◇◇◇◇◇◇◇◇◇◇◇◇◇◇◇◇◇◇◇◇◇◇◇◇◇◇◇◇◇◇◇◇◇◇◇

The problem is many family caregivers don't think they need the break. They feel like they are okay and can push through the tired feeling. Some even feel guilty for taking a break for themselves. But not only do you deserve time to rest, but you also need it to thrive.

When we started caring for my dad, I soon realized that I couldn't get to the beauty shop whenever I wanted, to church, or even to dinner with friends. Most of my regular weekly activities were interrupted because I had to spend what used to be my free time caring for him.

I didn't think much of it at first. I felt this was what I had to do for my dad and family. He gave so much to me. The longer I pushed through working a full-time job then coming home to care for him, the more the stress and tiredness pressed down on me. I didn't take the breaks as I should have because I didn't understand their importance at the time. Now I realize the importance of respite and the need to be rejuvenated. I want to make sure you know how to find or create a respite for yourself.

A respite is not a specific activity. It's a means of making sure you are taking care of yourself so you can care for your loved ones. Understanding respite is first recognizing that your duty as a family caregiver is its own job. When working for any employer, you are guaranteed specific break times. Sometimes that comes as a day off work, vacation days, lunch breaks, etc. Companies and the labor unions understand that working you for long hours without a break makes you a less effective employee. Your new job as a caregiver requires that you give them your full commitment and to make sure you can keep up with that level of responsibility. You must be mentally, physically, emotionally, and spiritually strong and stable. That means you must take time to care for yourself too by taking breaks and giving yourself time to repair.

I don't have any particular formula to tell you what that looks like because your rest is yours to define, but here are some examples to get you started:

◊ Spa day
◊ Learning how to balance finances
◊ A nap
◊ Waking up early and exercising
◊ Walking
◊ Going to the doctor for a checkup
  (or making sure your appointments are up to date)
◊ Seeing a movie
◊ Meeting with your lawyer
◊ Reading a book
◊ Remembering your favorite color
◊ Sitting having quiet time
◊ Gardening
◊ Going out with friends
◊ Church
◊ Getting your makeup done.
◊ Shopping
◊ Going to a painting class
◊ Going to a support group
◊ Learning new information on caregiving
◊ Going on a vacation
◊ Going back to school or taking a new class
◊ Lighting a candle and enjoying the fragrance
◊ Practicing breathing exercises.

Respite is yours to create. You have to identify the things that give you rest, that help you focus, and that you need to help you care for yourself. Once you know what respite you need, take it. Your health and the health of your loved ones are depending on you taking care of yourself.

Accessing Respite

Many family members quit their jobs, retire early, or cut their work hours to become family caregivers. They take part in caring for their loved ones through assisting with their needs and making sure that their needs are met. Usually, respite is taken through a home health agency, hospice agency, or some type of program that offers breaks (respite) to caregivers. Many of these programs depend on a payor source or other stringent requirements. If you don't have any of those things or meet the criteria, then you may not have access to respite from a program standpoint.

DISCLAIMER: There may be other avenues or programs being created right now to access respite that I don't know about. I want you to know that YES respite comes from all those sources. If those sources are not available, you will need to think outside of the box to get breaks and fill the gaps.

Gaps in Care

As I've worked as an RN, the healthcare environment is ever-changing. Some of the available programs are now non-existent. Even though the program's need still exists, there may not be a program available to fit every need. This is what I call a gap in care.

A Gap in care is an unidentified need that exists in any service or plan. So just because you have insurance doesn't mean that it will meet all of your needs. Think of it as a big puzzle of a picture that you have never seen before. When you look at it, since you've never seen it before, you don't know where to start. You ask someone close to you - friend, family, or coworker - if they have seen this picture before, and right away, they tell you they have never seen it before either and don't know where to start to put it together.

Having a gap in care is extremely frustrating to the healthcare team too. It leaves a healthcare provider feeling like, "How in the world can I help them?" There seems like there is no way. This is just how a family caregiver feels when placed in this situation. They don't know where to start. Even though they have access to healthcare, they quickly find out that it does not meet all of their needs.

Creating Respite

My father later died, and I started Caregiver's Respite to assist caregivers in learning all they can about caregiving. Everyone's caregiving journey is different. I encourage participants to learn about anything that applies to their individual caregiving situation.

Going forward, we have to think outside of the box to find ways for caregivers to get breaks. The high stress of caregiving can lead to burn-out and we cannot afford to lose any family caregiver. I am challenging every person reading this book to start learning everything they can regarding the health care needs that affects their family member.

NOTES:

_____

_____

_____

_____

_____

_____

_____

_____

_____

_____

_____

_____

_____

respite • renue • relief • recess • reprieve • rest • breather • breathing space • downtime • hiatus • interruption • lay-off • letup • lull • recess • relaxation • relief • reprieve • truce • break • time • adjournment • breath • cessation • ten • deferment • delay • deliverance • discharge • ease • exculpation • five • forgiveness • halt • immunity • intermission • interval • leisure • pardon • release • stop • postponement • protraction • rest • stay • coffee break • time out • renue • relief • recess • reprieve • rest • respite • breather • breathing space • downtime • hiatus • interruption • layoff • letup • lull • cessation • ten • deferment • delay • deliverance • discharge • ease • recess • relaxation • relief • reprieve • truce • break • time • adjournment • breath • cessation • ten • deferment • delay • deliverance • discharge • ease • exculpation • five • forgiveness • halt • immunity • intermission • interval • leisure • pardon • release • stop • postponement • protraction • rest • stay • coffee break • time out • renue • relief • recess • reprieve • rest • respite • breather • breathing space • downtime • hiatus • interruption • layoff • letup • lull • recess • relaxation • relief • reprieve • truce • break • time • adjournment • breath • cessation • ten • deferment • delay • deliverance • discharge • ease • exculpation • five • forgiveness • halt • immunity • intermission • interval • leisure • pardon • release • stop • postponement • protraction • rest • stay • coffee break • time out • renue • relief • recess • reprieve • rest • respite • breather • breathing space • downtime • hiatus • interruption • layoff • letup • lull • cessation • ten • deferment • delay • deliverance • discharge • ease • recess • relaxation • relief • reprieve • truce • break • time • adjournment • breath • cessation • ten • deferment • delay • deliverance • discharge • ease • exculpation • five • forgiveness • halt • immunity • intermission • interval • leisure • pardon • release • stop • postponement • protraction • cessation • ten • deferment • delay • deliverance • discharge • ease • rest • stay • coffee break • time out • lull • reprieve • break • renue • relief • recess • reprieve • rest • respite

CHAPTER TWO

Are You a Caregiver?

A Caregiver is a person who provides physical, spiritual, emotional, or financial support to an ill, aging, or disabled loved one.

It never ceases to amaze me that many people caring for loved ones do not consider themselves caregivers. I just had a conversation with a young lady and out of the blue, I asked her about caregiving. We talked about her family for about 10 minutes. Where she stated that she was not a caregiver, but her husband takes care of his mother. When I asked her in what way, she said he cooks, helps her with her grooming, changes her diapers, and that his mother lives with them. I asked her again, are you a caregiver? She still answered, "No, I do not change diapers or cook for her. My husband does all of that. I just sit with her sometimes when no one is there. I also make sure that when she gets up, she does not fall. My husband cooks and sometimes I fix her plate." We talked and talked about all the daily tasks that they do to take care of his mother. I looked at my watch and 20 minutes had passed. I finally informed her that the things she does for her mother-in-law are some of the things that a caregiver would do. I told her that she is a family caregiver along with her husband.

Activities of Daily Living (ADLs) is a term used in healthcare to refer to people's daily self-care activities. ADLs are defined as "the things we normally do" for ourselves such as feeding, bathing, dressing, toileting, and grooming. Instrumental Activities of Daily Living (IADLs) are not necessary for fundamental functioning. They allow individuals live independently in a community. When you help a family member who is unable to complete any of these tasks on their own, you are a caregiver. Some examples of ADLs and IADLs include:

ADLs
- Assisting with personal care such as dressing, toileting, grooming, or bathing
- Cooking meals, setting up their plate, or feeding them
- Helping them transfer inside and outside of their home

IADLs
- Picking up prescriptions
- Running errands
- Taking them to medical appointments
- Managing finances
- Medication reminders
- Light housekeeping
- Helping with grocery shopping

In recent years, chronic conditions are on the rise, making care more complex. Many nursing tasks are being performed at home by the caregivers, such as:

- Insulin injections or other shots
- Peg tube feedings/feeding tubes
- Trach care/suctioning
- Breathing treatment/oxygen therapy
- Wound/ostomy care

DISCLAIMER: I have broken down each definition to simple terms. Please, if you have a loved one who has any of these things for care in-home, please get an understanding from your healthcare professional on the requirements of care. Either of these items, with the wrong care, can result in an infection, etc.. Safety is important. You don't want to cause any harm. It is especially important that you get an understanding on how to care for these complex nursing tasks.

When you hear that your loved one has a wound, trach, oxygen, tube feedings, or insulin, please be aware that these tasks need extra teaching to maintain their integrity and function. Your job as a family caregiver is to get an understanding of the specifics.

Insulin Injections or other shots

Diabetics can control their blood sugar in several ways. One is by oral medication. Another way is to take insulin. Insulin is a medication given through a syringe with a needle on it (injection). If a person takes insulin, they will be instructed on how to give themselves a shot of insulin. Insulin can be very deadly if given in the wrong dosage. Please reach out to your healthcare provider if you must give insulin. They will instruct you on how to give it safely.

Peg Tube Feedings/Feeding Tubes

Feeding tube[2] is any flexible tube passed into the stomach for introducing fluids and liquid food. These feeding tubes are artificial ways of feeding a person. It is usually given to a person who cannot swallow or digest food as we usually do. These feeding tubes can be placed directly in the stomach or other parts of your Gastrointestinal System. If a person has a feeding tube, please get instructions for care from healthcare personnel on how to use or maintain these tubes.

Tracheostomy (Trach) Care/Suctioning

Tracheostomy (Trach)[3] is the surgical formation of an opening into the trachea through the neck specifically to allow the passage of air. A person who has a tracheostomy usually has a trach tube put in to keep the airway open. The patient may have the tube in permanently or temporarily. Either way, the tube requires care and many times the patient will need suctioning to clear secretions from the trachea. If your loved one has one of these tubes, it is particularly important to get a clear understanding of the care of it. Normally, the care is given by a licensed professional. Your healthcare team should train the family caregivers how to care for it.

Breathing Treatment/Oxygen Therapy

Breathing treatments are given to a person for a respiratory (breathing) problem. The medication is usually given via a machine called a nebulizer. If you have one of these machines, usually your nurse or respiratory therapist will instruct you on how to use this safely. Oxygen therapy is usually given to a person who may not be able to have normal levels of oxygen themselves. A respiratory therapist from a home health company will provide setup and education.

Wound/Ostomy Care

Wound[4] is defined as an injury to the body (as from violence, accident, or surgery) that typically involves laceration or breaking of a membrane (such as the skin) and usually damage to underlying tissues. You can get a wound in a lot of different ways. Wounds can be pressure sores, sometimes referred to as bedsores. Wounds can be incisions from surgery. They can also be irritations on the skin or abnormal openings to the skin that do not heal quickly.

Wound care is used to prevent infection or further complications and to promote healing. What I want you to know is they require specialized care and that a doctor will always prescribe a care regime. Usually, a nurse will carry out the orders and show you how to care for it as well. Over the course of my nursing career, I have seen many people go home from the hospital with wounds and no instructions on care. This care is serious.

Please, if you don't understand how to care for a wound, reach out to your doctor immediately. They will let you know what is normal and what is abnormal in the healing process.

Ostomy[5] is defined as an operation (such as a colostomy) to create an artificial passage for bodily elimination. This opening is made on the body, as the definition states, it is the creation of an artificial passage for something draining or used to help the body in its normal waste elimination function. These types of surgical passages generally require an appliance or a bag in order to collect the drainage. This may be called an ostomy bag, and some consider it a type of wound care. If you or your loved ones have this type of bag or have had this surgery, please get an understanding on how to care for it. Sometimes it takes more than one explanation to get the right knowledge for care.

Do you see any daily activities that you help a loved one with?

Are there other tasks you help a family member do regularly?

Are you a family caregiver?

Types of Family Caregivers

There are two categories of Caregivers - Formal and Informal. Formal caregivers are the paid professional caregivers such as doctors, nurses, or therapists. Informal caregivers are ones who normally do not get paid to take care of their sick family member or loved one. Informal caregivers come from our family, churches, communities, etc. Now, there are ways that people can get paid to take care of their loved ones but for this book's purpose, we will still consider them informal. Throughout this book, I refer to them as family caregivers (informal caregiver) and they are the very reason I wrote this book. Informal caregivers come in many different forms depending on family situations and the care recipient's level of need, but here are the main three:

Primary caregiver is usually the caregiver who is there on a regular basis many times they assist with daily activities and are incredibly involved in the decision-making process. They are usually the first representative that formal caregivers reach out to for information and feedback. They play a big part in advocacy and daily care needs.

Secondary caregiver is a caregiver that aids in other ways than the primary caregiver. They are usually used in the care that is not needed on a regular basis, or other care needs such as doctor visits, running errands, and financial concerns. They also support the primary caregiver as a backup.

Long-distance caregivers are caregivers that usually live 50 plus miles from the care recipient. If you live an hour or more and travel to care, you are a long-distance caregiver. Because of the distance, they depend on others to carry out most of the daily caregiving duties. Many deal with some guilt because of their inability to be present for most of the care recipient's needs.

Throughout my journey to help support family caregivers, I have found one of my main challenges was helping families understand the who, what, when, and how of family caregiving. I would say that about 20% of the time we support people who self-identify as caregivers, but 80% do not think they are a caregiver. Most people think the same as the lady mentioned earlier, believing that if they do not play a significant role in the recipient's care or their loved one can still do some tasks on their own, then they are not really caregivers. Another reason why caregivers sometimes do not self-identify is relationships. We feel that being obligated to someone because of our relationship to them means we are not a caregiver. We are just doing what we are supposed to do!

Husband/Wife Relationship

"I would take care of my spouse anyway, so that doesn't count."

Adult Child/Parent Relationship

"They took care of me, the least I can do is take care of them."

Parent/Adult Child Relationship

"This is my child; I'm supposed to take care of them."

A caregiver can be old or young. Many adolescents help primary caregivers to care for their loved ones. There are seniors taking care of their even older parents. Many caregivers work while others quit their jobs or retire early. Many families can find themselves in a caregiving role overnight and do not have the first clue about where to start.

NOTES:

_____

_____

_____

_____

_____

_____

_____

_____

_____

_____

_____

_____

_____

_____

_____

_____

_____

_____

_____

_____

respite • renue • relief • recess • reprieve • rest • breather • breathing space • downtime • hiatus • interruption • lay-off • letup • lull • recess • relaxation • relief • reprieve • truce • break • time • adjournment • breath • cessation • ten • deferment • delay • deliverance • discharge • ease • exculpation • five • forgiveness • halt • immunity • intermission • interval • leisure • pardon • release • stop • postponement • protraction • rest • stay • coffee break • time out • renue • relief • recess • reprieve • rest • respite • breather • breathing space • downtime • hiatus • interruption • layoff • letup • lull • cessation • ten • deferment • delay • deliverance • discharge • ease • recess • relaxation • relief • reprieve • truce • break • time • adjournment • breath • cessation • ten • deferment • delay • deliverance • discharge • ease • exculpation • five • forgiveness • halt • immunity • intermission • interval • leisure • pardon • release • stop • postponement • protraction • rest • stay • coffee break • time out • renue • relief • recess • reprieve • rest • respite • breather • breathing space • downtime • hiatus • interruption • layoff • letup • lull • recess • relaxation • relief • reprieve • truce • break • time • adjournment • breath • cessation • ten • deferment • delay • deliverance • discharge • ease • exculpation • five • forgiveness • halt • immunity • intermission • interval • leisure • pardon • release • stop • postponement • protraction • rest • stay • coffee break • time out • renue • relief • recess • reprieve • rest • respite • breather • breathing space • downtime • hiatus • interruption • layoff • letup • lull • cessation • ten • deferment • delay • deliverance • discharge • ease • recess • relaxation • relief • reprieve • truce • break • time • adjournment • breath • cessation • ten • deferment • delay • deliverance • discharge • ease • exculpation • five • forgiveness • halt • immunity • intermission • interval • leisure • pardon • release • stop • postponement • protraction • cessation • ten • deferment • delay • deliverance • discharge • ease • rest • stay • coffee break • time out • lull • reprieve • break • renue • relief • recess • reprieve • rest • respite

CHAPTER THREE

How Do I Start?

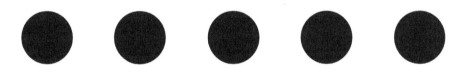

Many families can find themselves in a caregiving role overnight and do not have the first clue about where to start!

In my career, I have seen so many patients and family members who have been pushed into bad situations with their health. Sometimes it is very overwhelming - new diagnosis, tests that they don't understand, medications, therapies, and to top it all off, their life changes. They can't normally do what they used to do or even take care of themselves. This is hard on anybody when they must live differently because of an illness. This usually affects the whole family, not just the patient. When the family member becomes a caregiver, they ask me, "How do I start?" You start by getting organized.

Get Organized

Start by writing down everything you know about the person. It may seem elementary, but I promise that you will be dealing with many situations that will ask for a large amount of personal information. I have helped a lot of caregivers who have had all the wrong information about their loved ones. Case in point, I had a family member call me because the insurance company would not talk to them without their mother's social security number. Well, it turns out the social security number that they were giving them was the wrong number. They were distraught because they had no way of finding out the right number because they lived out of town.

It pays to double-check even the simplest of information that you have on your family is correct.

Examples of information you will need:
- ☐ Legal name (check against the Birth Certificate)
- ☐ Date of Birth (check against the Birth Certificate to make sure it is correct)
- ☐ Photo driver's license or any photo ID
- ☐ Insurance cards and discount cards
- ☐ Social Security number (check against the card)
- ☐ Church address and Pastor's name
- ☐ Funeral home (usually there is one that the family may prefer to use)
- ☐ Allergies (to food, medicine, etc.)
- ☐ Power of Attorney (notarized and officially filed)
- ☐ Weight, height, BMI - if available
- ☐ All medical information (even if you think it is not essential)
- ☐ Medicines (including dosage and frequency)
- ☐ Next of kin (with updated contact information and addresses)
- ☐ Family phone numbers (home/cell) and current addresses
- ☐ Account log ins and passwords
- ☐ Financial planner
- ☐ Companies or private individual they use for care
- ☐ Bills/Credit (and their usual payment methods)
- ☐ Medical equipment that they use/have
- ☐ Long-term care insurance or any insurance policies
- ☐ Wills or Trusts

- ☐ Support systems (Friends, Neighbors, Soror or Fraternity brother, Co-workers, church members, etc.)
- ☐ Marital status and Marriage Licenses (old and current)
- ☐ Death Certificates (of spouse/children)
- ☐ Recent tax returns (this may be important to know for income requirements or transitions to other levels of care)
- ☐ List of Properties (need to know when transitioning the level of care)
- ☐ Bank statements (of all accounts including Retirement and Annuities accounts)
- ☐ Veteran Benefits (if they - or their spouse - is a Veteran, find out their military status)
- ☐ Birth Certificate (try to find the original or one with an official seal on it)
- ☐ Organ Donor card
- ☐ Immunizations (look for the official records. If you cannot find them, start with the most recent flu and pneumonia shot record)
- ☐ Repairmen/contractors
- ☐ List of doctors/specialists (write the contact information on every doctor they have ever been to. See if you can find out the last time that they were seen.)
- ☐ Lab test results (latest results or any)
- ☐ Dental records (if any)
- ☐ Special diets
- ☐ Religious healthcare restrictions
- ☐ Religion
- ☐ Hearing and vision information (including prescriptions for glasses or hearing aids)
- ☐ Recent hospitalizations

- ☐ Their attorney's contact information
- ☐ Representative payee information
- ☐ Medicare/Medicaid number (check against the card)
- ☐ Employer name, phone numbers, email address, and physical address
- ☐ All previous addresses or other addresses lived
- ☐ P.O. Box location and rental information

Next, write down everyone that you think may help you take care of your loved one. You may start with family, but don't stop there. Your church, neighbors, friends, etc. It can be anyone not just your family. **THINK OUTSIDE THE BOX.**

Meet with his/her doctor

Meeting with the doctor can help you clarify some of those things that your family member said that never made any sense. Learn about what his/her condition is.

You may have to play catch up. Many times, if a person is going to the doctor alone, you may be uncertain about what exactly the doctor said to them. I remember when my father used to go to the doctor by himself, I would ask, "Daddy, what did the doctor say?" His responses were always good, never bad. Once, he told me the doctor said he could stop taking one of his medications when actually the doctor said that he needed to stop taking the milligram that he had been taking. His dosage was being lowered but he was not to stop taking the medication altogether.

Exercise Health Literacy

Health literacy refers to how a person can get the health information and services they need and how well they understand them.

As a caregiver, it's becoming more and more important to exercise health literacy. Health literacy refers to how a person can get the health information and services that they need and how well they understand them. It is also about using the information to make good health decisions.

Have you ever been confused by the medical terms and jargon health care professionals use? Health literacy can give you the skills necessary to become fluent in communicating effectively with your healthcare providers. The healthcare industry is continually changing. A caregiver must work hard to develop their communication skills just like an athlete would train. It takes consistency and training.

As a registered nurse, the number one barrier I have observed is that patients may not know what questions to ask. They usually depend on their healthcare professionals to give them all the information that is needed. These days you must be your own "navigator" in the healthcare system, and this is a skill you must develop in order to become health literate.

A primary strategy of health literacy is using 'plain language'. This strategy can be used by health care professionals, patients, and caregivers. Plain language takes complex health information and breaks it down.

When communicating with a healthcare professional, remember these critical points concerning plain language:

1. Ask the healthcare provider to organize and breakdown the information into understandable terms.

2. Ask the healthcare provider to provide you with the next steps you should take.

3. Write down the steps so you have an easy to retrieve record of the conversation.

Below are more steps to make sure of your success on your next doctor visit.

Four things to know when communicating with your healthcare professional.

1. Be Prepared. Most Doctors have a lot of patients, so their time is short. Have your questions ready. If you aren't present for the MD visit and someone has to take your place, consider typing your questions so they are easy to read. Have any paperwork that is needed ready to hand to the doctor.

2. Delegate a particular person to do the talking. Some people are well versed and have better communication skills, so utilize that person to help you understand what the doctor is saying. If you are a new caregiver, I highly recommend this. What I mean is, if you don't have knowledge of some medical terms, then the physician's words can go over your head. You can be easily intimidated and not get your questions answered. It is okay to bring someone with you to help you through the visit (see above Health Literacy).

3. Do your homework! It is vital to understand what is going on with your loved one. Therefore, please get familiar with some of the terms you heard your doctor say before, such as medication names and types of tests, and what they do before you go to the visit. This will help you follow along with your healthcare professional. It helps you beforehand. Don't worry about how you will get the understanding. JUST GET IT. Have your provider write on your medication bottle what the drug is for if you think you may get confused on what each medication does.

4. Be Ready. Be ready to tell the story. Sometimes you must get your provider up to speed on the past few weeks and the things that have gone on with your loved one. The best way to do this is to write things down. Write down symptoms, behaviors, dates, and times so that you have supporting dialogue to help paint the picture of what's going on with your loved one. You also can write down how the person has been feeling, how they are eating, and if they have been able to sleep. Make the doctor aware of any weight loss or gain as some medications and treatments can cause this.

● ● ● ● ● ● ● ● ● ● ●
You are their Advocate!
Defender against Opposition,
Supporter, Fighter, Spokesperson.

● ● ● ● ● ● ● ● ● ● ●

Caregivers are personal advocates for their loved ones. Without you, there is no one to fight for them. Good communication is critical with anyone, especially your doctor. Use good eye contact, keep calm, and remain confident. Your doctor is part of the team. Make up in your mind that you are not going to be intimidated, especially if you don't get the answers that you want from the doctor the first time. Be persistent and continue to ask questions until you get the answers you need.

Believe me when I say. It is a fight to keep someone that is sick well. Please be aware that to fight means to use strategy. Think of this book as a strategy to quickly start gaining your ground to be a successful caregiver.

NOTES:

respite • renue • relief • recess • reprieve • rest • breather • breathing space • downtime • hiatus • interruption • lay-off • letup • lull • recess • relaxation • relief • reprieve • truce • break • time • adjournment • breath • cessation • ten • deferment • delay • deliverance • discharge • ease • exculpation • five • forgiveness • halt • immunity • intermission • interval • leisure • pardon • release • stop • postponement • protraction • rest • stay • coffee break • time out • renue • relief • recess • reprieve • rest • respite • breather • breathing space • downtime • hiatus • interruption • layoff • letup • lull • cessation • ten • deferment • delay • deliverance • discharge • ease • recess • relaxation • relief • reprieve • truce • break • time • adjournment • breath • cessation • ten • deferment • delay • deliverance • discharge • ease • exculpation • five • forgiveness • halt • immunity • intermission • interval • leisure • pardon • release • stop • postponement • protraction • rest • stay • coffee break • time out • renue • relief • recess • reprieve • rest • respite • breather • breathing space • downtime • hiatus • interruption • layoff • letup • lull • recess • relaxation • relief • reprieve • truce • break • time • adjournment • breath • cessation • ten • deferment • delay • deliverance • discharge • ease • exculpation • five • forgiveness • halt • immunity • intermission • interval • leisure • pardon • release • stop • postponement • protraction • rest • stay • coffee break • time out • renue • relief • recess • reprieve • rest • respite • breather • breathing space • downtime • hiatus • interruption • layoff • letup • lull • cessation • ten • deferment • delay • deliverance • discharge • ease • recess • relaxation • relief • reprieve • truce • break • time • adjournment • breath • cessation • ten • deferment • delay • deliverance • discharge • ease • exculpation • five • forgiveness • halt • immunity • intermission • interval • leisure • pardon • release • stop • postponement • protraction • cessation • ten • deferment • delay • deliverance • discharge • ease • rest • stay • coffee break • time out • lull • reprieve • break • renue • relief • recess • reprieve • rest • respite

CHAPTER FOUR

Building Your Team

Another important reason I wrote this book is that I want people to begin to think proactively instead of always being in reactive mode when it comes to caring. If you have parents, they will age. If you have neighbors, church members, and people who you love, they will age and eventually need assistance and care. 10,000 people every day are turning 65. People are living longer. Have you looked at insurance policies? Many of them have changed the payout age to 121 when it used to be 100 years old, but they know that people are living longer. There is no way around it. What is wrong with preparing for it? Do you think if you prepare yourself for it that you are giving up? That you are giving them permission to get sick? That you are speaking things into existence? No, you are just being aware. Covid has taught us that you don't have to get sick or older to need care. So, let's talk about things that you can do proactively.

Team Players

Caregiving is not something that you can do alone you must develop a team. Building a healthcare team may be difficult for a family caregiver but try to think of it as something that must be done to achieve a goal. In order to develop any team, you have to:

1. Identify the players
2. Know what each player will be doing.

This works the same for caregiving. Each person has a

certain thing to do to help you achieve the goal. The goal is to care for your loved one. Please keep in mind everybody does not have to do the same thing to be a team member. Also, remember that if everybody on the team does not have the same goal, they might not be the best person for the job. Some caregivers might start off in one role but may not continue in the role.

One of the young ladies that I helped needed assistance with her brother. His care needs were that he needed 24-hour supervision, assistance with his ADLs, medication management, and sometimes he could not feed himself. He was not able to take himself to the doctor or communicate with the healthcare team. The caregiver knew that she was good at one thing so that's when we started developing a team. She was particularly good keeping track of his finances but needed help with everything else. Her goal was to take care of her brother at home so she started interviewing caregivers that could take care of his ADLs. She found him some transportation and she also found him a Nurse Practitioner that also made house calls.

Depending on your goals for your loved ones, you must:
◊ Know what their care needs are (ADLs)
◊ Know what kind of care different providers offer
◊ Match up the need to the care - some agencies provide non-licensed care (sitter and home maker services). Some offer licensed services such as home health and hospice.

Now, the two categories of caregivers are formal or informal. Keep in mind, you need both on your team. Informal caregivers come from our family, churches, etc. as we learned about in Chapter 3. Formal caregivers are the paid professional caregivers (see below).

Formal Caregivers

Doctor is a licensed medical professional. May be a general practitioner or have a specialty in an area. He or she is the one responsible for the management of any medical or wellness intervention. They are the ones who give the orders to other licensed professionals (such as those below) who then carry out the work.

Nurse (NP or FNP) is licensed as an advanced practice Registered Nurse with more years of education. They work under a medical physician's supervision to provide your care. Many people see nurse practitioners now instead of doctors as they are widely used in places that years ago only doctors were.

Registered Nurse (RN) is a licensed medical professional that performs duties such as doing assessments, giving medications, implementing treatment plans. She/he may come to the home through a home health agency or be in a hospital, clinic, or nursing home. Sometimes the RN is known as a 'Charge Nurse'. They can carry out the orders from the doctor or nurse practitioner.

Licensed Practical/Vocational Nurse (LPN or LVN) is a licensed medical professional that works under the RN to care for patients. She/he may come to the home through a home health agency or be in a hospital, clinic, or nursing home. They can carry out the orders from the doctor, nurse practitioner, or registered nurse.

Social Worker (SW) is a licensed member of the healthcare team who connects people with resources and coordinates help. Some are also trained to provide counseling.

Physical Therapists (PT) work with patients to get them stronger if they have had any weakness or injury to their body.

Occupational Therapist (OT) is a licensed person helping to strengthen a person who has had a surgery or injury causing a deficit in their ability to perform basic living activities.

Speech Therapist (ST) is a licensed person who helps patients to develop in any therapy related to the vocal cords and swallowing.

Respiratory Therapist (RT) is a licensed person who provides respiratory treatments, ventilator management, and oxygen therapy.

Certified Nursing Assistant (CNA) is a non-licensed – but certified – person who assists a patient with activities of daily living (or ADLs).

Personal Care Assistant (PCA) is a non-certified, non-licensed person who helps with home making services including some ADLs, light housekeeping, and light meals.

Lawyer is a licensed legal advocate. One thing people look at across the board and respect is when a person has all their business together. It is the same for a caregiver. If a caregiver has all their legal documents in order, then he/she is viewed as being savvy and prepared. If you are a new caregiver. I want to encourage you to meet with a lawyer as soon as possible and just talk to them about the legal aspects of caring for someone.

Some care will be provided from you and some will be provided by your family members. All the licensed and non-licensed care agencies require a payer source. If there is no payer source more than likely the team will be coming from your family, yourself, your neighbors, or your church members. All the care does not have to come only from you or your immediate family. Please keep in mind your goal is to build a team and get your loved one the care that is necessary.

Asking for Help

Asking for help can be a difficult task for anyone. Keep that in mind when dealing with the sensitive task of caregiving. This can be incredibly stressful for the care recipient. Independence is not something you give up easily. The person needing care sometimes will be embarrassed that they need some help now. Family caregivers can begin to expect a need for assistance to come even if the love one never specifically asks for help. When people ask for help it usually means that they have accepted a change in their condition. Acceptance does not always come quickly. In the normal grieving process, the acceptance usually comes last. As a family caregiver you will have to not only be aware of a need, but you will also need to define that need so a person can get the care that is required.

Let's talk about things that you can do proactively!

I went over who the formal caregivers are, now I want you to know that the formal caregivers come into your homes to interact with you only if they have a payer source. Meaning that these agencies in registries are businesses and they will help you for a fee. No nurse comes out to your house for free. No doctor sees you for free, Home Health does not come to your house for free.

There may be rare instances that you may see a formal caregiver at no charge - yes it does happen - but on the everyday normal side they come out and see you and expect some type of payment. Usually this is through insurance or other sources of payment. The proactive way of looking at this is that you should know what type of payer sources or insurances your family member has. You need to know this now if you can.

What will you be doing to prepare for that day?

When you are taking care of your love one in the home, know that if the level of care changes, you may have to change where they get their care. I have been doing this for several years, but I have yet to find a program that does 24-hour care except for a nursing home or your own home.

Has your loved one ever told you jokingly, "Do not put me in a nursing home"? And you say, "No, I wouldn't put you in a nursing home." Well, let me ask you what would you do? If a person says that to you then you need to start planning for their care. You need to know what it looks like. Nursing homes are places where people can get 24-hour care who cannot care for themselves. They usually need this care for safety reasons. They cannot be left alone, and they cannot dial 911 if they needed help in case of emergency, or they do not have someone there to stay with them to help them. This person may need 24-hour care. *What will you be doing to prepare for that day?*

NOTES:

_____

_____

_____

_____

_____

_____

_____

_____

_____

_____

_____

_____

_____

_____

_____

_____

_____

_____

_____

_____

_____

_____

_____

_____

_____

NOTES:

_____

_____

_____

_____

_____

_____

_____

_____

_____

_____

_____

_____

_____

_____

_____

_____

_____

_____

_____

_____

_____

_____

_____

_____

_____

respite • renue • relief • recess • reprieve • rest • breather • breathing space • downtime • hiatus • interruption • lay-off • letup • lull • recess • relaxation • relief • reprieve • truce • break • time • adjournment • breath • cessation • ten • deferment • delay • deliverance • discharge • ease • exculpation • five • forgiveness • halt • immunity • intermission • interval • leisure • pardon • release • stop • postponement • protraction • rest • stay • coffee break • time out • renue • relief • recess • reprieve • rest • respite • breather • breathing space • downtime • hiatus • interruption • layoff • letup • lull • cessation • ten • deferment • delay • deliverance • discharge • ease • recess • relaxation • relief • reprieve • truce • break • time • adjournment • breath • cessation • ten • deferment • delay • deliverance • discharge • ease • exculpation • five • forgiveness • halt • immunity • intermission • interval • leisure • pardon • release • stop • postponement • protraction • rest • stay • coffee break • time out • renue • relief • recess • reprieve • rest • respite • breather • breathing space • downtime • hiatus • interruption • layoff • letup • lull • recess • relaxation • relief • reprieve • truce • break • time • adjournment • breath • cessation • ten • deferment • delay • deliverance • discharge • ease • exculpation • five • forgiveness • halt • immunity • intermission • interval • leisure • pardon • release • stop • postponement • protraction • rest • stay • coffee break • time out • renue • relief • recess • reprieve • rest • respite • breather • breathing space • downtime • hiatus • interruption • layoff • letup • lull • cessation • ten • deferment • delay • deliverance • discharge • ease • recess • relaxation • relief • reprieve • truce • break • time • adjournment • breath • cessation • ten • deferment • delay • deliverance • discharge • ease • exculpation • five • forgiveness • halt • immunity • intermission • interval • leisure • pardon • release • stop • postponement • protraction • cessation • ten • deferment • delay • deliverance • discharge • ease • rest • stay • coffee break • time out • lull • reprieve • break • renue • relief • recess • reprieve • rest • respite

CHAPTER FIVE

Types of Care Providers

Now let's do a deeper dive on types of providers. A person can receive care in multiple places. The care is usually done by any of the team members we talked about in Chapter 4 and can be received in multiple locations. As a family caregiver, you need to understand the types of providers that provide care in locations other than your home. Every type of provider that we talk about you will need them on your team even if you don't presently need that level of care. I'm trying to say that you need to proactively develop a relationship or visit these types of facilities now before your love one actually needs it. If you wait until they actually need it, you will be overwhelmed on how to make this type of decision.

Case in point, I have provided nursing care in many different areas. One job that I had was a transitional care nurse in a hospital. We would have meetings every day for each patient on what they would need upon discharge. Some would be going home, and others would be going to sub-acute health care facilities. The hospital is an acute care facility. But if a person needs rehab, they would not stay in the hospital, they would go to a rehab facility. The social workers at the hospital would be in contact with the family and ask them what facility or rehab location, etc. they wanted their loved one to go to. Many times, the family member would not know which facility was best for their loved one. Often, the social worker would say or give them three choices of facilities in their insurance network. They would encourage them to go visit and look at the facility.

You will not have a lot of time to make up your mind when the hospital calls regarding a potential discharge date. You will need to move fast on some decisions. Let me tell you, these are not fast decisions to make, but you will have to make them fast. Proactively, it would help if you started developing relationships with the available resources now. Starting to look, call, and visit the facilities will help offset your future fears. Check them out before you even need them.

The world has had so many challenges to overcome. COVID-19 has been a game-changer for family caregivers. No longer are you able to go to the hospital with your loved one or go into long-term care facilities. Most of the communications that you, as a family caregiver, have is on the phone. That is a challenging aspect to grasp when you are the main person needed to answer questions about your loved one.

Several of my clients have reached out to me to let me know that the hospital has called them to let them know that their family member would not make it and recommend them to be placed on hospice. The person on the other side of the phone call needed them to decide immediately. That is why I am saying you should not wait until you need hospice to learn about hospice. Putting a person on hospice care is one of the hardest decisions that you will make. Learning and understanding Hospice will enable you to make an informed decision regarding your love one's final needs. As a family caregiver, you must get as much information as you can about anything and everything that will affect your loved one's care.

||||||||||||||
Proactive: *learn now.*
Reactive: *learn when you need it.*
||||||||||||||

Now don't get me wrong, you can't learn everything that you need to know in one day. Some things you will learn as you experience them. However, I am here to tell you that there are many things you can start gathering now. Remember when I mentioned that your loved one might say jokingly, "Don't put me in a nursing home?" Well now I am challenging you to start your learning process today. The following information will assist you in understanding the differences in the types of care providers.

Residential Care

Nursing Home is a facility that cares for patients who need around the clock care and supervision. They offer total care for the residents, many of which cannot care for themselves. Nursing homes provide both skilled and unskilled care, respite, and some rehab services. Medicare, Medicaid, Long-Term Care insurance, and veteran benefits are usually the way to pay for a nursing home. They also have private pay residents.

Care Home is a residential home for a senior or a disabled person that offers lodging, meals, and assistance with daily activities. Usually, the home is not very large and only houses a small number of people. They are generally in a residential neighborhood. Most of the people that live in the home only need assistance with some things - mostly their IADLs and some ADLs (see Chapter 2) - they are not total care patients. Many care homes are private pay. Also, depending on the city and state you live in, care homes may be called by other names. Keep in mind that the key to identifying care homes is that they mainly take private pay residents.

Assisted Living Facility is a residential facility that provides more of a monitored care to a patient. Most residents can take care of some of their ADLs and may receive some assistance. Usually, medications and meals are given to them. Some assisted living facilities have dementia or Alzheimer's units where there is more supervision and monitoring. Most accept private pay and some Medicaid.

I've only covered three of the most popular residential places where a person may receive care, but there may be more.

||||||||||||||

Proactive: *learning health literacy.*
Reactive: *learn as you go.*

||||||||||||||

In-Home Care

Sitter/Companion Care Services are agencies with non-licensed personnel who come in and perform various services around activities of daily living (ADL) needs. Most are private pay. Some Medicaid programs also provide these services.

Home Health Agency is a service that requires a doctor's order. These agencies send out licensed personnel such as Registered Nurses, Licensed Practical Nurses, Physical Therapists, Occupational Therapists, Speech Therapists, and Social Workers. These agencies accept payment through Medicare, Medicaid, and veteran benefits.

Hospice Agency/Hospice Houses are agencies that provide end of life care in several ways. One way is through palliative care. Palliative care supports a person's symptoms if the illness they have has no cure. Hospice will provide end of life care from a team of providers within the hospice agency. Some of the things they provide include medication, bereavement care, counseling, nursing, and some equipment. Hospice Houses are usually residential facilities that allow the family to participate in an atmosphere of care as the person transitions. Hospice care is usually paid for by Medicare, some Medicaid, and some private health insurance plans.

Adult Daycares are facilities where patients can come during the day and have activities to get them out of the house. These facilities are mainly for people with dementia. They are usually paid for through Medicaid, private pay, grants, and some veteran benefits. Some transportation services may be available depending on the facility.

IIIIIIIIIIIIII

Proactive: *plan for your family/parent's care today.*
Reactive: *learn as you're in it and overwhelmed.*

IIIIIIIIIIIIII

Learn what a person's insurance will cover. Going to the next level of care depends on the payer source. Now, what you would need to do as you care for your loved ones is find out what type of insurance they have and precisely what it will pay for and what it won't. Some insurances don't pay for home health, rehab, equipment, and some medications. Find out now instead of later if you can.

NOTES:

respite • renue • relief • recess • reprieve • rest • breather • breathing space • downtime • hiatus • interruption • layoff • letup • lull • recess • relaxation • relief • reprieve • truce • break • time • adjournment • breath • cessation • ten • deferment • delay • deliverance • discharge • ease • exculpation • five • forgiveness • halt • immunity • intermission • interval • leisure • pardon • release • stop • postponement • protraction • rest • stay • coffee break • time out • renue • relief • recess • reprieve • rest • respite • breather • breathing space • downtime • hiatus • interruption • layoff • letup • lull • cessation • ten • deferment • delay • deliverance • discharge • ease • recess • relaxation • relief • reprieve • truce • break • time • adjournment • breath • cessation • ten • deferment • delay • deliverance • discharge • ease • exculpation • five • forgiveness • halt • immunity • intermission • interval • leisure • pardon • release • stop • postponement • protraction • rest • stay • coffee break • time out • renue • relief • recess • reprieve • rest • respite • breather • breathing space • downtime • hiatus • interruption • layoff • letup • lull • recess • relaxation • relief • reprieve • truce • break • time • adjournment • breath • cessation • ten • deferment • delay • deliverance • discharge • ease • exculpation • five • forgiveness • halt • immunity • intermission • interval • leisure • pardon • release • stop • postponement • protraction • rest • stay • coffee break • time out • renue • relief • recess • reprieve • rest • respite • breather • breathing space • downtime • hiatus • interruption • layoff • letup • lull • cessation • ten • deferment • delay • deliverance • discharge • ease • recess • relaxation • relief • reprieve • truce • break • time • adjournment • breath • cessation • ten • deferment • delay • deliverance • discharge • ease • exculpation • five • forgiveness • halt • immunity • intermission • interval • leisure • pardon • release • stop • postponement • protraction • cessation • ten • deferment • delay • deliverance • discharge • ease • rest • stay • coffee break • time out • lull • reprieve • break • renue • relief • recess • reprieve • rest • respite

CHAPTER SIX

Things Can Change

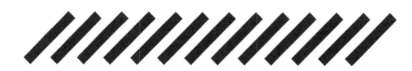

So, now as you are caring for your loved one, you have some things in place and have built up confidence in caring. I think that is awesome! But please be aware that things can change.

Level of Care Changes

One of the major things nurses learn is assessment skills. Assessment starts as soon as we walk into a patient's room. We look at the person physically and assess their position, skin, color, how they are breathing, what they are saying, how they say it if they respond slow or fast and if they are sleeping or awake. We are observing their surroundings for hazards and odors also. We are looking for changes and anything abnormal. As a family caregiver, you will be looking for sudden or subtle changes in the loved one you are caring for from their current normal. For example, if they are walking, an abnormal for them would be them limping. If they are limping, an abnormal would be them unable to walk. If they are already unable to walk but they can move their hands, an abnormal for them would be if they could not move or use their hands.

///////////////////////////

When the care needs change, you have to change the way you care.

///////////////////////////

While taking care of my father, one of my family members (who had a stomach virus) came over to the house.

Within 8 hours, my dad started having a lot of diarrhea and became dehydrated. We took him to the hospital where he received a lot of fluid to correct his dehydration. Since he was older, he could not tolerate so much fluid at once and soon became overloaded with fluid. Prior to going to the hospital, he was alert, able to talk and move around. The fluid that he received made him short of breath, lethargic, and unable to express himself. When I saw this, I realized that even though he was sick and elderly, things had changed. When the doctors looked at him, they thought he was just old and getting ready to pass, but I let them know that he did not come in with shortness of breath and the other changes. He only came in for a stomach virus and diarrhea. My assessment of his changes helped bring a quick response from the medical team because I knew him. Caregiver, what I want you to know is that as you spend time with your loved one, you will know their normal. Be confident when you see a change and know that it is a change. Be persistent in communicating the change to your healthcare provider and your family. Sometimes family may be some of the hardest people to convince of changes.

What does a level of care change mean to family caregivers? When things change from their normal it means that your care changes from the normal. As we continued to take care of our father, he went through so many levels of care changes in one year that it threw us for a loop. Every month we were doing something different to care for him.

When he first got sick, we could leave him for short periods of time. Then later someone had to be there at all times. When he first got ill, he could feed himself. Later we had to assist him more and more. When he first got ill, we were mostly supervising. Which later turned into doing everything for him. **When the care needs change, you have to change the way you care.**

The Decision of Care Making

Parts of being a caregiver are scary and uncertain. When you are dealing with making decisions for your loved one, sometimes you do not know what to do. Your heart is right toward them but sometimes you fear that the decision you have to make for them may be wrong. I promise this happens all the time. Normally, you would talk to the person that you are trying to make a decision for to include them in the decision-making process but sometimes you can't. The response that they give you may not be what is best for them. Sometimes if you have an aging parent or loved one, they lack the ability to think things through. This is not always the case, but it happens often. As our loved ones age, they need someone to help them make medical decisions. They need someone to help them think it through.

I remember talking to my dad, and I told him, "Pop, you know you have been getting sicker. How do you want us to care for you?" He responded, "I don't plan to need any care. I plan to beat this!" I continued to talk to him, but he did not give me anything to work with. He kept talking about other things. He would not accept the fact that he could not care for his personal needs. After that conversation, I honored his wishes by not trying to organize help for him and it literally stressed me out because I tried to do it his way.

The care that is needed does not always line up with what is desired. As a family caregiver, please listen to your loved one. Try to allow the care recipient to make as many decisions as they can but it is up to you, the caregiver, to know when to change to another level of care. You must make some decisions based on safety, need, and care for yourself.

Role Reversal

Role reversal can happen because a new set of duties are needed and therefore you have to set new expectations to meet your goal. If you are just used to being a daughter, the expectation may be different than being a daughter who is a caregiver. Because you have a new role, know that you don't have to do everything right. Everything won't be handled perfectly, and you will make mistakes. Learn from them, keep going and stay in control. Remind yourself of this because a shift in roles that has new expectations can weigh on you very heavily. You are not perfect, and this is new. Keep moving forward to make the adjustments needed in your new role.

I considered myself a great nurse, but I was not prepared for being a family caregiver. One thing that I realized was that even though my father was in his late 80's when he got sick, I was not emotionally prepared, and I had no plan for him. Realistically, what was I thinking….......? A man in his 80's?? I guess I thought he would live forever.

I never thought he would ever be sick and looking at it now, I had no plan for his care. I did not even know what he wanted. As I think back on this, the message that I want you to understand is that caregiving affects EVERYBODY. This is not an isolated concern. In this book, I talk about my father and caring for him at an older age, but anyone can become a care recipient at any age.

NOTES:

_____

_____

_____

_____

_____

_____

_____

_____

_____

_____

_____

_____

_____

_____

_____

_____

_____

_____

_____

_____

_____

_____

_____

_____

_____

_____

_____

_____

NOTES:

respite • renue • relief • recess • reprieve • rest • breather • breathing space • downtime • hiatus • interruption • lay-off • letup • lull • recess • relaxation • relief • reprieve • truce • break • time • adjournment • breath • cessation • ten • deferment • delay • deliverance • discharge • ease • exculpation • five • forgiveness • halt • immunity • intermission • interval • leisure • pardon • release • stop • postponement • protraction • rest • stay • coffee break • time out • renue • relief • recess • reprieve • rest • respite • breather • breathing space • downtime • hiatus • interruption • layoff • letup • lull • cessation • ten • deferment • delay • deliverance • discharge • ease • recess • relaxation • relief • reprieve • truce • break • time • adjournment • breath • cessation • ten • deferment • delay • deliverance • discharge • ease • exculpation • five • forgiveness • halt • immunity • intermission • interval • leisure • pardon • release • stop • postponement • protraction • rest • stay • coffee break • time out • renue • relief • recess • reprieve • rest • respite • breather • breathing space • downtime • hiatus • interruption • layoff • letup • lull • recess • relaxation • relief • reprieve • truce • break • time • adjournment • breath • cessation • ten • deferment • delay • deliverance • discharge • ease • exculpation • five • forgiveness • halt • immunity • intermission • interval • leisure • pardon • release • stop • postponement • protraction • rest • stay • coffee break • time out • renue • relief • recess • reprieve • rest • respite • breather • breathing space • downtime • hiatus • interruption • layoff • letup • lull • cessation • ten • deferment • delay • deliverance • discharge • ease • recess • relaxation • relief • reprieve • truce • break • time • adjournment • breath • cessation • ten • deferment • delay • deliverance • discharge • ease • exculpation • five • forgiveness • halt • immunity • intermission • interval • leisure • pardon • release • stop • postponement • protraction • cessation • ten • deferment • delay • deliverance • discharge • ease • rest • stay • coffee break • time out • lull • reprieve • break • renue • relief • recess • reprieve • rest • respite

CHAPTER SEVEN

Self-Care

■ ■ ■ ■ ■ ■ ■ ■ ■ ■ ■

I thought long and hard about putting this chapter in the book. Wellness (self-care) is not the first thought of many caregivers. Most of the time they don't give any thought to this. Some might say:

> » "I don't have time for this, I have to take care of my loved one."
> » "I will start tomorrow".
> » "I'm doing what's important today taking care of my loved one."
> » "They need the care more than I do".
> » "I'm okay."

When you mention self-care, it may offend them until they face their own health crisis. Think about it, if you are taking care of someone who has had a stroke and paralyzed on one side, do you realize that they are counting on you to fill their void of only being able to use one side? That means that you must have strength to cover their deficit. If you take care of someone who cannot speak clearly because of an illness as you spend more time with them, you begin to understand how they communicate. Wherever you go, people are counting on you to convey what they are trying to say. If you take care of someone who has lost their vision, that means that they are counting on you to see what they can't see. Without even asking, they are expecting your eyes to be good, your strength to be strong, your communication skills and mental capacity to be intact. You must take care of yourself as you care for your loveds one.

***You are not the best caregiver unless
you take care of yourself.***

The statement above now becomes relevant. Even
though there may be time and priority concerns, your
care is as important as theirs. Without you, who would
they depend on to see, to stand, and move forward?

As a caregiver, how do you start taking care of yourself?
Think of it like this - there are two things that you do in
life: (1) things you do for others and (2) things that you
do for yourself. For example, getting enough sleep does
a lot for your body. It allows your body to heal and repair
itself. As a family caregiver there are many challenges
that prevent you from getting enough sleep. Even though
that is true, we want to focus on the fact that everyone
needs adequate sleep so that they can function. Getting
enough sleep is what you do for you, but it also helps
you care for your loved one.

On a piece of paper make two (2) columns, on the left
write down the things you do for yourself and on the
right, write down things you do for your loved one. As
you fill this out, give yourself 2 points for each thing you
write down for yourself and 1 point for the things you do
for others. Reflecting on the statement above, if you take
care of someone who has a stroke, and they are weak on

one side they are counting on you to cover their weakness. Everything that you do for yourself it counts double to their one. Use this exercise to start looking at all the things you give out daily compared to what you give yourself. Is it equal?

If you give to others more than you give to yourself, you are headed down the wrong path. But it is not too late. You can start right where you are. You can begin with the awareness that you are a statistic when you start caring for your loved one. That means you are not the only one, and there is a whole category of individuals in similar situations. Many have already been where you are and learned the value of self-care and the consequences of ignoring yourself while caring.

Self-Care Strategy

I heard a caregiver say that when she took care of her loved one, she took care of herself. She said she didn't have a lot of time, but this is what she did. She would get this bag and take it wherever she went as she cared for her dad. This bag was packed JUST FOR HER! In her bag were a set of knitting needles, yarn, gossip magazines, water, snacks, a picture of exercises, crossword puzzle book, fragrant lotion, and her phone. The magazine represented mindless activity. She stated, "Sometimes I want to get away for a minute." She would look at those magazines and they would lift the weight of caring from her mind. She loved gossip, but you may love magazines with beautiful homes or travel magazines to help you visualize somewhere else. The snacks she put in the bag had dual roles. They were things that she loved to eat and things that were good for her. She had different kinds of popcorn in the bag as well as unsalted almonds. She had regular and flavored water along with sugar free candy and cookies.

When she had to be sitting in a doctor's office for a while, she would pull out her knitting needles and yarn. This was her true hobby that she did not have to give up. Sometimes they would have to wait on the doctor so long, that before you knew it, she would have knitted a whole hat! When she used the lotion, the fragrance helped her mood when things didn't seem so positive. It made her feel happy. The phone represented her Facebook family. She was able to communicate with others and would not feel the weight of isolation. Occasionally, she would pull out the card with the exercises on it. She would look at it and stretch just like the person in the picture did. Impromptu sessions of exercise and stretching kept her feeling mobile.

Stress and Caregiving

Caregiving can be one of the greatest opportunities that a person can have. Giving care and showing concern to anyone can be extremely rewarding. It can also be incredibly stressful.

Stress is one of those things that come with the job. The main way to deal with it is to acknowledge that caregiving may be stressful and try to find ways to manage the stress. You could be prone to isolation. When you start caregiving, you might not have as much time on your hands to do for yourself as you used to so sometimes it causes you to change the way you socialize. Many times, in caring for someone else it can cut into your sleep pattern making you more irritable. It can also cause a financial burden on the household. You will also find that sometimes worrying about your loved one can captivate you because something you want to change you cannot change. Many times, you feel like you are losing that person and may start a type of grieving process: denial, anger, bargaining, depression, and acceptance.

As you care for your loved one, please be aware that unmanaged stress can leave you angry, irritable, sad, and fatigued. Here are some other symptoms of stress:

- Changes in weight
- Pain
- Headaches
- Eating more or less
- Anxiety

One of the main roles of a family caregiver is to provide emotional support. You are helping your loved one to cope with what is going on with them. You are becoming a full-time listener as they vent about their circumstances. You listen and encourage them that everything will be okay even though you know that it doesn't always work out that way. As you become an emotional cheer leader, it also can leave you needing emotional support as well. It can also be emotionally draining if you are caring for a love one and your relationship is not the best. This puts a strain on your caregiving. You will have to put your differences aside as you accept this assignment. If you cannot this may affect how you care.

Make sure you find ways to support yourself emotionally. Get help. Join a support group (a group of people who can relate to a situation or problem). This is a wonderful tool for a family caregiver. When you join a support group you will be around like-minded individuals who are going through the same things that you are going through. There is no judgement. Many times in caregiving, when you get around others you will find that they may have a solution to a problem that you are facing.

Prolonged stress that is not managed can lead to depression. Depression can lead to loss of hope and discouragement. You may feel tired all the time or have thoughts of harming someone or yourself. Get help - talk to your mental health professional right away to see if you suffer from depression or any mental condition. The sooner you are aware of your condition, the better outcome you will have.

Ways to Minimize Stress and Get Respite

Stress happens and depression is possible. One of the ways to minimize stress is to get away from your situation. You must do this often. Do not leave your loved one if you think you need to be there at a certain time. However, you must get away for a break so you can renew your thinking and your actions whenever you can.

Try to have some 'me time'. That statement can mean so many things to a person. Not sure what that looks like? Try one of these:

☐ Get a massage.

☐ Get on YouTube and learn a relaxation technique.

☐ Soak in the tub. Now you may not be able to do it long, but even 10 minutes sometimes helps with your day.

☐ Continue the organizing process. Nothing would be more stressful than to get someone to care for your loved one while you're gone, and they can't find anything that they need.

- ☐ Go walking. If you can't leave the house, walk in place.
- ☐ Spray some perfume. When you smell good you feel good.
- ☐ Take time to journal. Sometimes you must write down what you are feeling to get it off your chest. Once you write it down let the feelings and emotions stay in the journal and not in your mind.
- ☐ See if someone will give you a break for 2 hours to sleep (NAPTIME).
- ☐ Learn a new skill. Find a hobby online, something that you can do without leaving the house.
- ☐ Listen to music.
- ☐ Dance or sing.

Every time I do a consultation with a new caregiver, I let them know they are a statistic. Their situation has been evaluated and observed from many different angles by people all over the world. People have studied the results and found both positive and negative outcomes. Your caregiving journey is already statistically defined by aspects like your health, wealth, and social behaviors. Those possible outcomes are already studied, but your own final outcome can be buffered with strategy and the negatives offset with self-care and planning.

Love yourself! Know that this journey does not have a master blueprint, you are making it up as you go. It is okay if you make a mistake: learn from it, keep going, and pat yourself on the back. I dare you to hug yourself and let yourself know that you are doing a great job.

NOTES:

_____
_____
_____
_____
_____
_____
_____
_____
_____
_____
_____
_____
_____
_____
_____

NOTES:

NOTES:

_____

_____

_____

_____

_____

_____

_____

_____

_____

_____

_____

_____

_____

_____

_____

_____

_____

_____

_____

_____

_____

_____

_____

_____

_____

_____

_____

_____

1. AARP International. (2019). *The Aging Readiness and Competitiveness Report: United States.* Retrieved July 1, 2019. **https://arc. aarpinternational.org/countries/unit-ed-states**

2. Merriam-Webster. (n.d.). *Feeding Tube.* In Merriam-Webster.com dictionary. Retrieved September 30, 2019, from **https://www.mer-riam-webster.com/dictionary/feeding%20 tube**

3. Merriam-Webster. (n.d.). *Tracheostomy.* In Merriam-Webster.com dictionary. Retrieved September 30, 2019, from **https://www.mer-riam-webster.com/dictionary/tracheosto-my**

4. Merriam-Webster. (n.d.). *Wounds.* In Mer-riam-Webster.com dictionary. Retrieved September 30, 2019, from **https://www.mer-riam-webster.com/dictionary/wounds**

5. Merriam-Webster. (n.d.). *Ostomy.* In Mer-riam-Webster.com dictionary. Retrieved September 30, 2019, from **https://www.mer-riam-webster.com/dictionary/ostomy**

Made in the USA
Columbia, SC
15 July 2021